Yoga
by Chanel Diamond

Table of Contents

1. Introduction

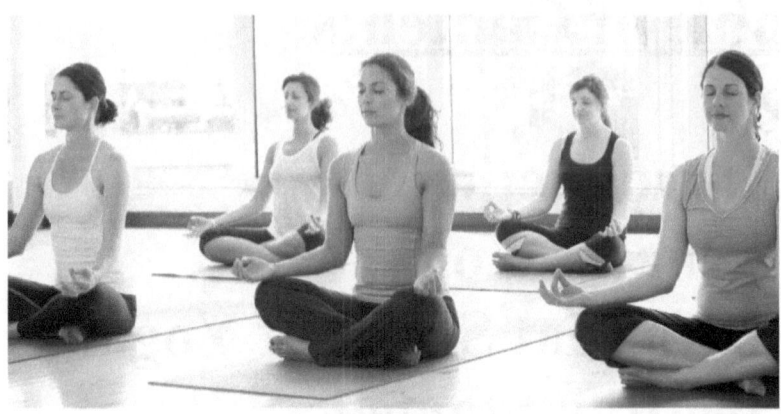

The body needs a natural lifestyle and other basic conditions like an adequate nutrition, exercise, inner harmony and some other energetic qualities to maintain its health and vitality. Your earthly body is constantly interchanging information with your thoughts, emotions and reactions. Anything that is manifested in your body is a reflection of the unbalances in your life.

This tradition assures that your body is simply a material manifestation of your subtle energies and that it's a vehicle to move around in this material world. You know what philosophy I'm talking about? It's yoga.

The word yoga comes from a word in Sanskrit that means union, and it's not a coincidence that is named like this. Yoga is a tradition, a discipline, a philosophy and a lifestyle that bonds your material, spiritual and mental being.

You see, every human being has a body with which they can reach spiritual realization and gradually reach higher levels of consciousness. Yoga is a preventive and healing tool that allows you to be healthy and reach your maximum potential. Yoga helps you develop and become the true you; yoga is intuition, yoga is a universal thought, yoga is balance and yoga gives you inner peace. Yoga offers a holistic approach to health, and considering that both, body and mind are inseparable this is the best method to achieve a perfect state of well-being.

Yoga works on your body, transforming all your cells with its Asanas, and techniques and by doing this automatically your mind and your spirit are transformed too. Yoga creates balance between your mind and your body. This millenary practice is capable of changing your nervous system through its series of Asanas, Pranayamas and meditations; working in the whole you and not focusing only in your body or only in your mind.

In this book you'll learn all that you need to know about yoga; its benefits, its purpose and philosophy. This book is also a complete step-by-step guide that will help you get started and master many postures and breathing techniques.

You will discover a whole new and exciting world. You will be amazed with what your body can do and how good you feel once you begin practicing yoga. You will also learn that everyone can practice yoga, and that the more you get into it, the better you will feel.

All the benefits in all aspects of life that this discipline can bring you are impossible to mention or cover completely and some others are just impossible to describe with words. Yoga is a system, but more than that it's an individual experience. There are millions of reasons of why you should practice yoga; I can't mention them all but I can assure you that you will never regret this big step you are taking. You will know what life without stress is and how it feels like to be totally conscious and alert. If you practice all that is instructed in this book I guarantee you will feel wonderful and will look even better. Yoga revitalizes your mind and your spirit, it enhances all the systems of your body, making them perform at a top level, and the results are truly amazing.

Yoga is a complete exercise that will give you everything you need. You will work on your body; you will look thinner, toned and beautiful. Yoga, will also give you something that most of other exercise workouts won't and simply can't give you: inner peace. Join me in this journey and enter this fantastic world of millenary traditions, mysteries and secrets. You will forever be thankful with yourself that you did!

2. What is Yoga?

Yoga is a system that helps develop your physical, mental and spiritual potential. It helps reach optimal health and overall wellness. It's a word that means "union" in Sanskrit; yoga sees union between your body, mind and spirit. Yoga philosophy assures we are connected, that we are one with everything that exists and that we all have the qualities of the universe: love, wisdom and plenitude.

Yoga is for Everyone

Yoga looks for unity between human beings, is tolerant and universal. It goes beyond cultural, social and religious differences. Yoga has a transcendental sense because it's spiritual but not religious or dogmatic. Yoga is related with the nature of the world, with the essence of humans and the sense of life. You can go as deep as you want to go; you can only practice techniques for physical health or you can search for inner growth and transformation. Yoga doesn't tell you how to live or in what to believe, you take what you like and practice what you want. Yoga is freedom, and yoga sets you free.
Yoga is for everyone; anyone can practice yoga because it's a universal training that looks for health and happiness. This is why yoga has diverse forms, schools and practices. This amazing philosophy adapts to people. There are different types of yoga for different types of bodies, for moments of life, physical states, beliefs and cultures.

Yoga = Health

Some people think that yoga is a new trend, but yoga has been around for over 5000 years. The postures are only a part of this discipline and some of these postures are stretching exercises that are fundamental for having good health. The stretching makes you more flexible over time, but also, expands your inner self and allows you to be more connected with the universe and live a happier a life. Yoga postures mean strength, balance, knowledge and energy that translate in a symbolic way into your life. Yoga works in your body in order to be able to reach your mind and the "superior you". Yoga is a tradition about integral development and includes different practices such as meditation, breathing exercises, relaxation, positive thinking, attention, self-consciousness and ethical life.

Many people practice yoga for many reasons; to have more vitality, to reduce stress or anxiety, to feel good with their bodies. Others practice yoga to augment mental faculties, to treat physical ailments or to conserve good health. Many people claim that it helps them sleep better and with back pain. The truth is yoga helps with all this and many other deeper and more profound things, as maintaining peace in moments of change and transformation. It helps with depression, to overcome fears, it makes feel more passion for life, boosts confidence and self-esteem, it gives more sense to one's life; it makes you grow spiritually. People that practice yoga often feel freer, braver and just…phenomenal.

Yoga is Fun

Yoga is very entertaining and is a constant process. With yoga you learn how to maintain balance, how to stand on your hands and turn your head up-side-down. You bend, you stretch and it's exciting to see the changes in your body and abilities every day. With every posture, you guide your body to new possibilities. Every day you will be amazed of how relaxing your mind and expanding your body can change the view you have towards everything. In a short time you'll notice how yoga extends to all your life. What happens is that it integrates the mind and body in a regular exercise that doesn't force or extenuates you, it doesn't judge or compete. Yoga is pleasant instead of been tortuous, it's loving and not aggressive and is the entrance to a whole new and fantastic world that will change your life forever. Yoga is a constant work in yourself that will never end, because you are eternal, infinite.

Yoga Sets You Free

Yoga sustains that radiant health and happiness are your birthrights. In this sense, yoga is the liberation of mental conditionings that have separated you from your true nature. Yoga is a path with many dimensions that will help you find your real essence again. Yoga doesn't give you anything; it allows you to see what you already have. Yoga helps you free yourself and releases everything that is not good for you. It helps explore the magnificent potential of your body and your mind to make them transcend. Yoga makes you plentiful, beyond the limited notion of "I" and allows you to experiment the luminousness of the union with the universe. Even though it is referred to as a discipline, its finality is not to achieve or fulfill anything because everything you need you have it already in you.

Yoga is Unity

We live in a time where almost everyone has a strange relationship with their body. People care more about their image than anything else, but have no clue of how to really take care of their body. People don't listen to their bodies, are not in tune with its necessities, its processes, its possibilities. No one provides the correct breathing, food, stretching or exercises the body needs. Of course almost no one considers the importance of inner serenity or positive thinking for the cells, organs and material being to form an integral unity. People have a notion of the body as a machine that is disconnected from the mental and emotional aspects of life. People tend to believe they don't have any saying over their body and don't see health as a natural state and as the result of a balanced life. Everyone sees medicine as an artificial treatment that is required only when diseases appear and never stop to wonder why they are sick in the first place.

Yoga has a holistic concept of the body, of the entire being, mind and spirit that make part of a perfect unity. Yoga says we are all universal beings, interconnected to everything and everyone. Through the stillness of mind you can identify with universal consciousness; that is your true essence. This state of consciousness is what yoga is.

3. Different Styles of Yoga

The style of yoga you come close to the first time is crucial for you to connect with tradition. It makes a big difference in the moment of having a particular experience. Not all yoga practices are the same; not even in a same tradition.

There are many styles of physical yoga and many other forms of yoga (not all are physical), so you have many options to explore. You have to find the best style for you; one that adapts to your body, needs, wants and objectives.

In this book we will mainly focus on the Asanas (postures), of physical yoga that comes from Hatha Yoga, but you'll also learn Pranayama (breathing techniques). There are moments in which you will prefer a more mystical and devotional practice, one in which the physical work is exigent and others in where the practice is softer and meditative. Your body and your spirit will ask for what they need and with time you will learn to listen to them. There's no better style than other, as long as yoga doesn't lose its essence, all practices bring enormous benefits.

Yoga, even with its diverse methods has improved many lives and health states. As you dig deeper into this philosophy you'll find that you will feel more attached to a certain style. This is completely fine; just don't forget that yoga has as a central component: expansion, so stay open to new possibilities.

Combining different styles of yoga can give more variety to your practice, and the truth is that no matter what methodology you are using, you will never stop evolving. You will feel better every day; every time you practice you will improve your physical, mental and spiritual health. A time when yoga it's not an effort, but a necessity will come, and you will ask yourself, "How could I live without yoga before?" Further on you will understand what I'm talking about, yoga is so fantastic that becomes a part of your essence.

Yoga is not always the same

The answer to this question is yes and no. Yoga in its essence obeys a same tradition, shares a common purpose of spiritual realization. However, its big history, the encounter with other philosophical and religious traditions, among other factors such as adaptation to western culture has caused yoga to diversify in different branches. Some of these are classical and other traditional, but they all seek the same: physical and spiritual wellness.

All that I mentioned above has provoked the separation of the different elements that form Raja Yoga (ethical guidelines, meditation, breathing techniques, concentration, postures, integration). This is the cause that some teachings focus only on some instructions and ignore others, and also the reason that people often think that yoga is only a system of exercises and postures. In reality, all of these are only a line of one type of yoga; Hatha Yoga.

Hatha Yoga

When yoga is mentioned in a generic sense, generally it's making reference to a very specific aspect of the yogic tradition: physical yoga. Within the broad spectrum of elements that form this philosophic and scientific system, the practice of Asanas (postures in Sanskrit), sequences, breathing and Mudras have a particular name: Hatha Yoga.

The origin of the word "Hatha" is a good starting point to explain what this style of yoga consists in. It's a lot more powerful, spiritual and deeper than you can imagine. The reaches it has go beyond a simple system of exercises. Hatha could be traduced as force or will, in a sense related to the body and everyday life. Hatha Yoga strengthens the body and will; it's a discipline that requires commitment, but also increases the capacity of equanimity and of listening to the wisdom of universal consciousness. It's a path to explore the potential of the body and mind.

Hatha has another meaning, and it's indispensable to mention it to understand the real meaning of yoga. "Ha" means sun and "tha" means moon. Hatha Yoga is the yoga of the opposites and balance. For this reason, it brings strength and lightness to the body and thoughts. It combines our feminine and masculine aspects; exercise with stillness; action with intuition; the physical and the subtle; our right brain hemisphere with the left; reestablishes the connection between mind and body; balances the excess and deficiencies of the chakras.

When we talk about Hatha Yoga we are referring to almost all the practices of physical yoga that are defined with other names: Vinyasa, Anusara, Ashtanga, Iyengar, Sivananda and Kundalini among others. The difference between one another is that they can include various modern adaptations of Hatha Yoga. They all make emphasis in determined aspects of this classical yoga or incorporate new elements of other philosophical traditions. Some consist in more specific postures and sequences derived from Hatha Yoga. In other words, Hatha Yoga is the most authentic of the physical yoga techniques and its more traditional form.

Hatha Yoga is a paused and generally soft practice. It consists in traditional positions, coordination, deep and conscious breathing. Hatha Yoga is a practice based in meditations in which the attention is constantly attracted towards the present moment, the language of the body and to the space between the eyebrows. This form of yoga also includes the practice of Pranayama (exercises to control breathing), relaxation, Mantras and meditation. Hatha yoga is an excellent introduction to yoga because it constitutes the fundamentals of this discipline.

This style of yoga is a spiritual work that begins with the body, because body, according to the yoga tradition, is the vehicle through which we live and reach spiritual evolution. Hatha Yoga also constitutes a marvelous healing method, a system for longevity, for quality of life, improves mind and body's health, gives inner peace, confidence and provokes the expansion of the heart. Its virtues are infinite, and this is why more people get into this discipline every time.

4. Getting Started

By now you already know what yoga is, what benefits it brings to your overall health, and you also know that Hatha Yoga is an excellent way to start in this discipline. Now, we will go through some important points before throwing ourselves into the practice of different techniques and postures.

To begin with, you have to maintain a fresh vision at your present and open your heart. This is the first thing to do; remember that according to yogic tradition, this is the natural state of your being. What we call yoga are techniques that will help free yourself of what has separated you from the magnificent state of unity. Instead of generating resistance to life, you have to be able to see life with clarity and accept it just as it is. This is not called passiveness; is about creating a space for wisdom and action instead of reaction. If you expand you align with existence, you flow. When you are feeling closed, your mind or what we call ego, interposes with your old beliefs and the eternal paradigm between good and bad clouds your senses. You have to learn that things simply are. So first, start with observing your inner processes. Watch your thoughts, judgments to yourself and to the rest of the world; watch your negative emotions. When you do this, you start creating consciousness of what you really think and of who you really are. Try to see every instant as something new, and whatever you do, do it with love; this is the first step to practice yoga. From here on, you will enter a different world; you will be transformed, healthy, you will feel radiant and plentiful.

Practicing Yoga

The main characteristic of physical yoga is that it's centered in Asanas. These postures generally are stretching exercises, and also include some balance, strength and relaxation training. There are positions in where you are standing and others were you are seated or inverted. Sometimes you bend and other times you twist and spread. To form these Asanas you need to have plain conscious on the movement or the stillness. This means you have to be completely immersed in what you are doing. You have to forget about everything else, it's only you at this moment. Bring complete attention to your body, its sensations and rhythms. You have to focus in your breathing; this will fill you of vital energy and will free your physical and emotional knots and hindrances. When practicing yoga, thoughts are only to be observed, without judgment or attachment. If for some reason you get distracted or your mind starts wandering around, always bring it back to the moment you are at; to the present. Yoga is a meditation that seeks to integrate the body and mind; it seeks a balance between happiness and stillness. When you practice yoga you are calmed but full of clarity and energy. Your main goal has to be to blend the spirit and the body, to activate vital energy and to achieve inner silence to be able to connect with your essence.

What You Need to Practice

For original Hatha Yoga you only need your body and a present mind. Generally simple and comfortable clothes are more than enough, there's no need to buy anything special or spend fortunes in fancy garments. You will also need yoga mat, or if you don't have one, you can use a blanket where you can practice. Bare feet, an open mind and heart are also requirements. You have to be willing to nourish your body, to relax your mind and to elevate your spirit. If for some reason you don't have mobility or you think you are not flexible and you believe you can't practice Asanas (postures), you can still do yoga. You can start with the meditation, relaxation and breathing techniques, then your own body will ask for more. Even if you start slow, you will still have the amazing benefits as the loving attitude and will be more open to a compassionate and generous life. To be completely present and to be amazed with the greatness of life, to feel how you transcend your own self and turn it into a beautiful natural landscape is also yoga. There are many ways to practice yoga, because yoga is everything that brings you back to the state of integration with existence so don't worry, yoga is for everyone.

The main characteristic of Hatha Yoga is that it is paused, meditative and generally soft. It's a yoga that adapts to the majority of bodies and health states, and preserves the relaxing faculties of yoga while it promotes good health and elevates energy. It's essential that you find a space that vibes with yourself as well as it is essential that you begin with a basic level, something for beginners that guides you through every step.

In yoga there's no judgment, no competition, no comparisons, so there's nothing to fear. Just open yourself and allow the real you to come out, and then, just…let go. Don't worry if when you start you are a little stiff and clumsy, it happens to everyone at the beginning. After some time of practicing you will learn to love your body and to honor the process because yoga is not about getting somewhere, remember, you are already where you have to be and already have with you everything you need. You will learn to stop judging and to be compassionate with your own self; this is one of the most beautiful lessons yoga will give you. If you have fear to do something for the first time, but you still move forward and do it, is a signal that you are leaving behind the things you are comfortable with, the things you already know and are taking new challenges. When you do this you are growing spiritually. If you decide to practice yoga I can assure you one thing; you will thank yourself forever for taking this decision.

5. Yoga Breathing Techniques

Breathing is a primary and necessary function even though you are not conscious about it most of the time. When you practice yoga, this process becomes conscious and turns harmonious, balanced and pacific.

Each of the Asanas you will learn and practice further on will be accompanied by its correspondent breathing. When you manage to control your breathing, the rest will flow a lot easier because it influences directly over every emotional state. When you learn how to breathe correctly, you are brought back to your center, and you find your balance point.

What is Pranayama?

The word Pranayama in Sanskrit literally means "breathing control", and to be more exact the word "Prana" means energy and "Ayama" means creation. Pranayama is a science that works by manipulating your vital energy through different breathing techniques. This form of yoga has amazing effects over your physical, mental and spiritual states. It will give you vitality, clarity of mind and superior states of consciousness.

Before you start practicing Pranayama it's important you become familiar with your breathing, your lung capacity, the physical effects of an adequate breathing and the surprising relationship that exists between your breathing, your emotional states and your mind. It's also important that you notice of how valuable your breathing is in your everyday life.

As in any other yoga practice, these exercises require your full attention and presence. You can practice Pranayama anywhere because you don't need anything special. The ideal is that you find a place where you feel comfortable and relaxed and where you are not distracted. Try to disconnect with the rest of the world and silence your mind. This is a time for your development and your well-being; there's nothing more important than this.

Uro Pranayama

This breathing technique is performed with the intercostal muscles expanding through the thorax. This exercise can be done while you are sitting, but it will be a lot easier if you lie down. Make sure you are comfortable so you are able to focus on your breathing without anything else distracting you.

Exercise

1. Your attention should be focused on the thorax region, specifically in the ribs. Lift your hands and pose them gently over the upper part of the chest.

2. When you inhale, expand the thorax and raise your chest. Focus on the middle region of the chest. Imagine how the frontal, lateral and back parts of the chest inflate. Feel how your thoracic box expands.

3. Exhale the air completely.

4. To confirm you are doing the right movement, keep your abdomen slightly contracted to make sure you are breathing with your thorax and not your stomach.

Keep breathing like this six more times, counting every time you inhale and exhale.

Kuksa Pranayama

Kuksa Pranayama also called deep abdominal breathing, is one of the best breathing exercises because it brings air to the lowest and biggest parts of the lungs. This breathing technique has to be slow, profound and you have to use the diaphragm correctly. It permits to experiment the diaphragmatic breathing, purifies the organism and eliminates tension and calms anxiety. It's one of the most common Pranayama practices, and in this technique you have to focus on the abdomen.

Exercise

You can sit if you prefer, but I recommend you lie down. Make sure you are comfortable and don't allow anything to distract you.

1. Breathe in deeply through your nose filling the lower part of your lungs with air; this will provoke your belly to come out. Your stomach has to look completely swollen.

2. Close your eyes and pose your hands gently over your stomach. Focus on this zone of your body.

3. The smooth descent of the diaphragm gives your abdominal mass a soft massage. Little by little, the lower part of the lungs fills with air. Breathing has to be slow, relaxed and silent. If you hear yourself breathing, it will not have the desired effects; it means you are doing it too quickly. Inhale slowly, feel how your belly expands. Your chest should not move. Count to five when you breathe.

4. Exhale slowly the air through the nose and feel how your stomach flattens. Count to five when you exhale. It's important to empty the lungs completely, and to expel the most quantity of air possible.

When you have emptied the lungs completely, your abdomen will relax and the process starts all over again. It's essential that you inhale and exhale through your nose and also to maintain the stomach relaxed.

Anuloma Viloma

Even though you don't realize it, you tend to breathe in cycles of one or two hours; first one nostril prevails and then the other. Breathing through only one nostril for a long period of time can cause your energy to decline. Anuloma Viloma or alternate breathing is an ancient breathing technique that applies a profound soothing effect over the mind and helps you learn how to breathe in a balanced way. When you alternate your breathing the energies and the airways of the nervous system recuperate balance.

Exercise

Before you start, clean your nose with a handkerchief. Sit comfortably on a chair or in your bed with your back completely straight.

1. Rest your index finger in the space between the eyebrows and the middle finger over the palm of your hand. Now, put your thumb over the right nostril and your ring finger on the left nostril.

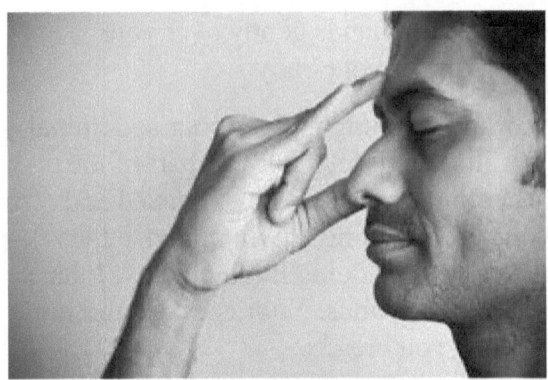
Anuloma Viloma Finger Position

2. Now close only the right nostril with the thumb. Inhale through the left nostril while you count to five.

3. Close both nostrils with your fingers while you contain your breath and count to five. If it bothers you, reduce air retention.

4. Without moving the ring finger, lift your thumb and exhale all the air through the right nostril counting to five. Continue, inhale through the right nostril counting to five. Retain air for five seconds.

5. Lastly, close the right nostril and uncover your left nostril allowing the air to come out only through the left side of your nose. As you exhale count to five and then retain air for five seconds.

Repeat the entire round four more times.

Ujijayi
Ujijayi or resounding breathing is a soothing technique that balances the nervous system and gives serenity and calmness to the mind and emotions. The sound it emits could be compared to the calming influence of the ocean. If you want, while you practice this breathing that expels vicious air from the lungs and that purifies the respiratory system, you can visualize the relaxing and peaceful ocean.
Exercise

1. Sit with your back comfortably stretched or lie down with your legs slightly open.

2. Exhale air thoroughly.

3. Inhale slowly through the nose until you fill your abdomen and the lungs with air.

4. Slightly contract the upper part of your throat while you exhale and inhale slowly through the nose. Emit a low whistle sound. The sound doesn't have to be loud but you have to be able to hear it.

5. While you inhale and exhale, keep breathing slowly, focusing on the sound you are producing.

Repeat this exercise three to five times.

Kapalabhati

Kapalabhati or head breathing is an invigorating and purifying breathing technique that literally means, "Lighting the skull". It airs the organism by notably augmenting the delivery of oxygen to the body. It tones muscles, the stomach, strengthens the diaphragm, increases energy and foments concentration. This activity produces a quick elimination of attached mucus in the respiratory system. It reinforces the nervous system, and allows absorbing significant amounts of oxygen. Kapalabhati aids in circulation and raises the metabolic performance.

In the psychic aspect it elevates the control over one's self and the capacity to focus. I advice that you don't surpass the duration of this exercise; if you don't follow instructions properly instead of feeling better you will provoke discomfort to yourself.

Exercise

1. Sit down with your back comfortably extended. Look at the floor and close your eyes.

2. Take a big breath in and exhale the air vigorously through your nose. All the air that you inhaled has to come out in one big blow. When you exhale, contract your stomach, do it as when you cough.

3. Once you release all the air, stop contracting your stomach as well. You will feel how without doing anything special, due to the relaxation of your stomach, your lungs will fill with air again.

4. Exhale vigorously again through your nose, only that this time you won't release the air in one blow. You have to do eleven short and energetic exhalations.

Kapalabhati is composed with eleven forced and interrupted exhalations. You only use your stomach to do the contractions, and the ribs should not participate actively during this technique. Try not to force your nostrils and larynx while doing this for best results. After performing the first eleven, rest for some moments and repeat the exercise only one more time. After fifteen days you can add another series of eleven; this means your routine will be of three series of eleven exhalations each.

Brahmari
The vibration this invigorating humming breathing technique causes is similar to the one that is created when singing the Om mantra. Brahmari helps eliminate tension and calms the body and mind. Focusing on the sound and vibration you produce allows you to live in the present, giving you peace and satisfaction.
Exercise
1. Sit comfortably with your back straight. Close your eyes and lower your gaze.

2. Inhale deeply through your nose counting to seven. If you want, you can change the count so that you feel comfortable.

3. Slightly open your lips and emit a humming sound while you exhale through your mouth counting to fourteen.

4. As the intensity of the humming augments, try to make your lips vibrate as you exhale through your mouth.

Repeat this exercise two more times.

Sufimata Pranayama

This breathing technique is also called Maternal Sufi Breathing and it foments the sensation of protection, security and support. As with other breathing exercises, the increase of oxygen produces an improvement on skin, cleans internal organs and promotes toxin elimination.

Exercise
1. Sit down with your back comfortably extended, or lie down with your legs slightly open.

2. Breathe through your nose counting slowly to seven and hold your breath until you count to fourteen. If you want you can modify the count to be more comfortable.

3. Exhale through your nose counting to seven. After you exhaled all the air, stop breathing during fourteen seconds.

Repeat this exercise several times.

Nadisodhana
Nadisodhana is a mix of the Ujijayi and Kapalabhati techniques. The purpose of this exercise is to clean and purify the channels of subtle energy, balancing the circulation of Prana. This is achieved by alternating the inhaling and exhaling flows between both nostrils. Before anything else, you have to learn "Prana Mudra" because this will be essential for this exercise.
Prana Mudra
Extend your hands and gently pose your index and middle fingers in the palm of your hand like in the picture below.

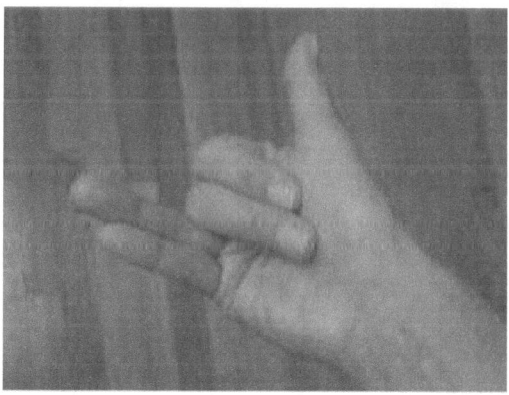

Exercise

1. Inhale deeply through your nose and exhale slowly.

2. Cover your right nostril using prana mudra.

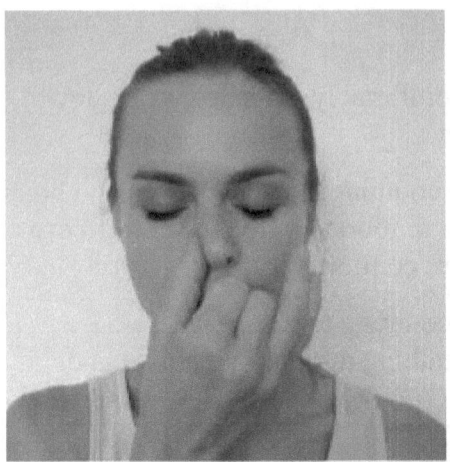

3. Inhale vigorously through your left nostril. Do this is as profoundly as you can, controlling your abdomen.

4. Without uncovering your right nostril, cover the left side of your nose with your ring finger and hold your breath for two or three seconds; fill your lungs with air.

5. Now, leave your ring finger in your left nostril (picture below) and exhale slowly and deeply all the air from your lungs.

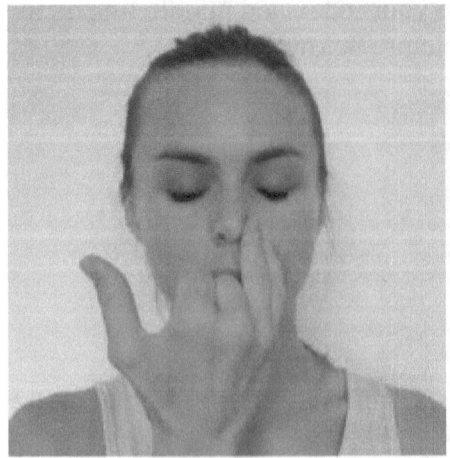

6. Suspend your breathing for about two or three seconds without air in the lungs.

7. Still covering the left nostril, inhale deeply through the right side of your nose. Control your abdomen as you do this.

8. Cover both nostrils again and detain your breath for two or three seconds with your lungs filled with air.

9. Now keep your right nostril covered and exhale slowly and deeply through the left side of your nose.

10. Suspend your breathing for about two or three seconds without air in the lungs.

Start all over again and repeat the whole process several times, always alternating between the two nostrils.

Kumbhaka

The Sanskrit word Kumbhaka means "voluntary retention of breath", and this is what this technique is all about. The physiology of air retention implies cardiac, circulatory and respiratory changes; all of them very important. In Kumbhaka, the breathing is detained after every inhale and every exhale between three, and twenty seconds for beginners. Experienced yogis can often hold their breath for several minutes!

The main purpose of these air retentions is to achieve a better conversion of air oxygen, and naturally, everything else that is derived from it. After a few seconds of holding your breath with the lungs filled with air, the respiratory center registers a change in the composition of blood. This change stimulates the spleen; contracting it and provoking it to throw enormous amounts of red blood cells into your blood flow. Also the body temperature elevates and the nervous system is relaxed.

When you breathe in a normal rhythm, your organism absorbs only 6% to 20% of the oxygen contained in the air you inhale. When you retain air, the time that oxygen is in contact with the lung membrane is prolonged, and this augments its absorption. Kumbhaka provokes significant modifications in your metabolism; the most important is the partial decomposition of sugar in blood.

Filled Lungs Technique

Retention with filled lungs is called Antara Kumbhaka.

1. Inhale through your nose deeply counting to seven.

2. Exhale through your mouth slowly counting to seven. Repeat this five times; breathing has to be slow and relaxed.

3. Next, you will inhale deeply through your nose counting to ten; suspend the respiratory movement with the lungs filled with air. Contain your breath for ten seconds.

4. Exhale the air out of your lungs slowly and continue breathing in a relaxed way.

Repeat this sequence four or five times. If your breathing is still comfortable, you can extend the time of air suspension. If after exhaling you notice you are suffocated, then relax and breathe normally until you can continue with the exercise.

Empty Lungs Technique

The retention with empty lungs is called Bhaya Kumbhaka and you should practice the technique with filled lungs before trying this one.

1. Inhale through your nose deeply counting to seven.

2. Exhale through your mouth slowly counting to seven. Repeat this five times; breathing has to be slow and relaxed.

3. Now, inhale deeply through your nose counting to ten.

4. Exhale slowly counting to ten and when your lungs are completely empty suspend the respiratory movement. Contain your breath for three seconds.

Repeat this exercise four or five times. If your breathing is still comfortable you can extend the time of air suspension for up to five seconds. If after a sequence you feel suffocated, breathe normally for a couple of minutes until you can continue with the exercise.

Paripurna Pranayama

When you are stressed you breathe in a quick and superficial way, and this only causes your stress levels to elevate. When you practice the complete breathing technique or Paripurna Pranayama, your emotions are soothed, tension is relieved, muscles are relaxed and you have better focus. This exercise purifies your respiratory system by expelling vicious air from your lungs and oxygenating blood cells. Breathing not only has a direct effect over the body's vitality, but is also related with psychic energy and mental health.

Before anything else you will learn the Sukhasana posture first.

Sukhasana

Sit on the ground or on a blanket and cross your feet like in the picture below.

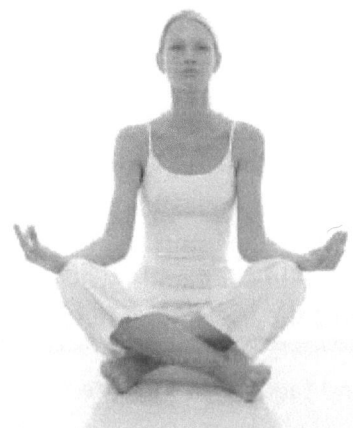

Now that you know Sukhasana, let's go on.

Exercise

1. Sit in Sukhasana position; breathe in deeply and then slowly empty your lungs.

2. Now inhale slowly through your nose but only breathing with your stomach; don't let your ribs move.

3. Without interrupting the air flow, continue inhaling through your nose. Elevate your inferior ribs and middle part of the thorax allowing the air to enter slowly through the center of your lungs.

4. As you feel the air coming in gently, and still inhaling elevate the upper part of your chest permitting the air to come in

through the lung apex. As you do this, slightly contract your stomach. All of these movements have to be done in a continuous way; one after another, forming one unit, without forcing anything at any moment. It has to be uniform, smooth and natural.

5. Now comes the exhaling. Start by losing the tension and air in the upper part of your body. Follow with the middle section and finish by releasing all the air from your stomach until it is completely relaxed.

Air has to flow through your nose in a regular, soft and uniform way. You can repeat this exercise from to up three to ten times in a single session, but if you are just starting, take it slowly. Begin with three sequences the first day and increase one every day.

Benefits of Pranayama
-Better blood oxygenation and toxic elimination.
-Better ability of the body to assimilate foods. Digestive organs, like the stomach, receive more oxygen and function more efficiently.
-Improvement of the nervous system, including the brain and nerves.
-Gland rejuvenation; mostly the pituitary and pineal glands. The brain benefits immensely because it requires the triple amount of oxygen than the rest of the organism.
-Skin rejuvenation; skin becomes softer and facial wrinkles are reduced.
-Through the diaphragm movements during these exercises the abdominal organs –stomach, intestine, liver and pancreas –receive a massage, and these massages stimulate blood circulation on these organs
-Lungs get active and healthy.
-Stronger and more efficient heart.
-Weight control; the extra oxygen helps get rid of fat.
-Mental relaxation. The states of the mind and the body are strictly related, and with more oxygen in your brain and body your mind receives the benefits.
-These exercises produce an augment in the lungs and thorax elasticity, creating an increase in the breathing capacity during the whole day, not just while you do the exercises.

6. Asanas - Step-by Step Guide

Tips To Start With

-Before starting with any Asanas is important you know the capacity your body has. Please, don't push your body into a posture and never cross your limits. Remember that yoga is not a competing sport; the progress can be slow, but with practice, dedication and time you will become flexible.

-Some poses affect your emotional state and energy in different levels. Some postures or sequences like" Saluting the Sun" and other standing positions are very invigorating, so it's better to do them only in the mornings. Forward inclinations, inversions and resting poses are more appropriate for night.

-Many of your everyday activities tend to pronounce the use of only some parts of the body. To be harmonious and to reach a healthy balance it's necessary to keep all parts of the body evenly strong and flexible. Always work with both sides at the same intensity and for the same period of time. For example, if you do forward bends, do them backwards too, always look for balance.

-Whatever is your purpose for practicing yoga, always stretch first. Every routine has to start with a good warm-up.

-After your warm-up you can then start with simple positions and then include other Asanas that strengthen your body and give you resistance.

-Your routine has to be balanced and should include poses from every group: stand, sit, bend, twist, work backward, forward, etc. Everything should be gradual, don't rush! Between every posture always take some minutes to breathe and relax.

-Passing from one posture to another is called a sequence; I will be giving you sequences you can start with after reviewing the basics.

-After every practice it's important you take at least ten minutes to relax your body. Relaxation is a complete receptive state where and through deep breathing your body can recover and rejuvenate itself. Always finish your routine with a relaxing pose.

-Consider yoga as a continuous process. Some people are less flexible or have stronger muscle groups, so please be patient and loving with yourself. Yoga is an activity for all your life, and persistence and discipline are necessary to receive all the benefits that it has to offer.

-Don't worry if in the beginning you cannot do the Asanas properly, I can assure you they will become easier with time and practice. The stiffness of your muscles will diminish little by little. Always start with the basic positions and when you feel comfortable, move to others that require more effort and elasticity.

-You don't need anything else but yourself to be happy. The time you dedicate to nourish your body and your spirit, focusing in your practice, been conscious, and experimenting the benefits yoga brings you, will help you find inner peace and be a balanced, healthy and happier person.

Stretching Exercises

If you have never practiced yoga before, it's probable your muscles are tight, and your joints are a bit stiff. With time and the lack of use of different parts of the body mobility is reduced, and it becomes harder every time to do certain activities. But, don't worry this is one of the many benefits yoga brings into your life. Yoga augments flexibility, and increases the capacity to stretch.

The first things we'll go through are some simple and easy stretching exercises that you need to do to warm-up. You don't have to do all of them, just choose the four or five you feel more comfortable doing. Remember to be patient and never go beyond your limits.

Standing Position –Stretching the Neck

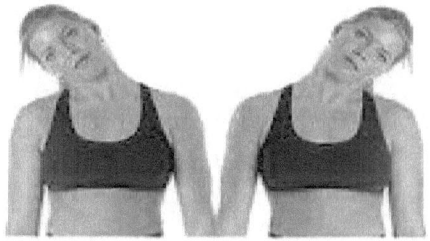

1. Stand up and place your feet width ways of your shoulders. Slightly contract your stomach and stretch your back. Put your shoulders down and keep your chin parallel to the floor.

2. Now, slowly move your head towards your right shoulder. Breathe in deeply through your nose and as you do this center your attention in the left back side of your neck. Maintain the position for five seconds.

3. Exhale through your mouth as you bring your head back to the center. Slowly move your head towards your left shoulder. Breathe in deeply through the nose and center your attention on the right back side of your neck.

Repeat this exercise two or three more times and always remember to contract your stomach.

Stretching the Shoulders

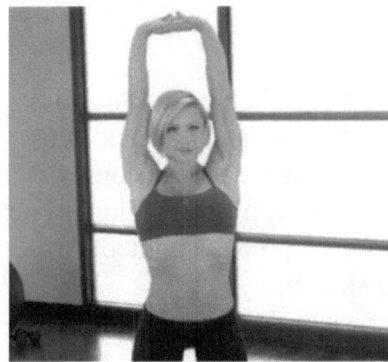

1. While you are sitting or standing, contract you abdomen and stretch your back.

2. By the sides, lift your arms on top of your head. Cross your fingers and place your palms looking towards the ceiling.

3. Breath in deeply through your nose counting to seven and exhale deeply through your mouth counting to seven. Breathing has to be quiet and comfortable. Center your attention in the shoulders and the arms.

4. Do at least five deep breathing rounds maintaining the position. If you can, try to keep your elbows at the side or behind the ears.

5. Gently put your arms down and repeat the whole sequence two more times.

Bent Over With Hands Behind

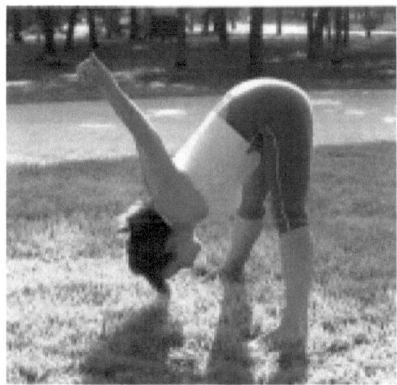

1. Stand up and spread your feet. Contract your stomach and stretch your back comfortably.
2. Cross your fingers behind your back. Slowly bend forward and as you do this inhale deeply through your nose.
3. Extend your hands and arms upwards and backwards, always keeping them straight. Hold the position for three seconds. Center your attention in your back and arms.
4. Still in the bending position, let go of your arms and exhale through your nose as you move back to a vertical positions.
Repeat this exercise at least five more times.

Shoulder Rotation

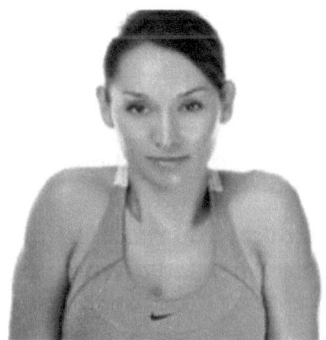

1. Stand up slightly spreading your legs apart. Contract your stomach and stretch your back.
2. Shrug your shoulders and then start a rotating movement backwards. Relax any tension you have as you move slowly your shoulders in circles.

3. Center all of your attention on your neck and shoulders. Your breathing should be relaxed and calmed. Do this for at least 45 seconds.

Standing Leg Stretch

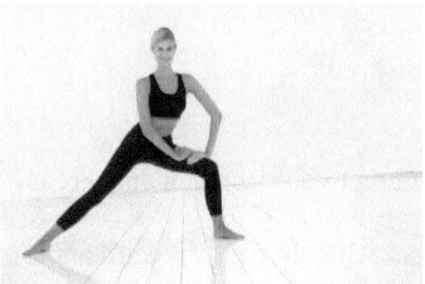

1. Stand up and spread your legs apart. Contract your stomach and extend your back.
2. Slightly bend your right knee and place both hands over your leg. Keep your back as straight as you can and tight your left leg muscles. Breathe in deeply through your nose and hold position for three seconds, centering all your attention in your left leg.
3. Slowly move back to an upright position exhaling all the air from your lungs.
4. Now, slightly bend your left knee and place both hands over your leg. Keep your back as straight as possible and tight the muscles of your right leg. Breathe in deeply through your nose and maintain position for three seconds centering all your attention in your right leg.
5. Move back to a vertical position and repeat the entire sequence four more times.
In this exercise, you have to move all the weight of your body from one side to another always contracting your stomach and giving support to your back.

Forward Bend

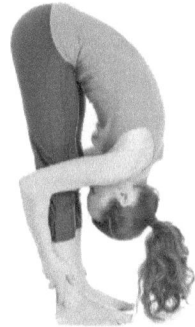

1. Stand up and spread your feet width ways of your shoulders. Contract your stomach and stretch your back.
2. Put your chin on your chest and bend forward as if you are trying to reach the floor.
3. Hold your elbows in front of you and use the weight of your body to stretch the back side of your legs.
4. Breathe in deeply through your nose and as you exhale push your elbows towards the floor. Center your attention in the back of your legs, feel how they stretch.
5. Now, still holding position, slightly bend your knees and after two seconds straighten them again.
6. Move back to an upright position always contracting your stomach. Do a shoulder rotation and breathe in deeply through your nose and exhale through your mouth.
7. Repeat the sequence but now don't hold your elbows; instead try to get hold of your ankles, stretching your legs and back. Maintain the position for ten seconds and repeat both sequences two more times.

Side Stretching

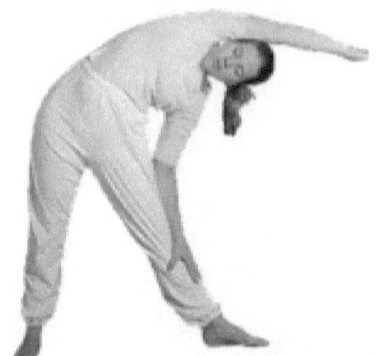

1. Stand up and spread your legs apart. Take a deep breath through your nose and exhale through your mouth.
2. Lift your right arm and pass it over the top of your head. At the same time slide your left arm through your left knee and hold position for at least three seconds.
3. Breathe in deeply through your mouth and center your attention in the right side of your body. Stretch your side as much as you can and remember to always contract your stomach.
4. Move back slowly to a vertical position and repeat exercise using the other side of your body.
Repeat the whole sequence four more times.

Hip Oscillation

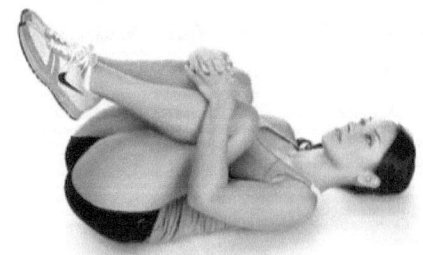

A. 1. Lie down on the floor and use a yoga mat or blanket to feel entirely comfortable.
2. Bring your knees to the chest and grab them firmly around the knees. Press your knees against your chest.
3. Every time you exhale move the knees towards your chest. When you inhale, you have to move the knees away from the chest.

4. Keep doing this movement and try to connect it with your breathing. Remember every time you inhale move the knees away from the chest and every time you exhale you move them towards your chest.

B. 1. Now, let go of your knees but keep them bent. Put your hands at your sides, near the hips with the palms facing the sky.

2. Inhale and extend your right leg and hold this position for three seconds.

3. Exhale slowly and bring back your leg to the chest. Do the same movement with your left leg and repeat sequence for three times.

C. 1. Bring your knees back to the chest, and this time try to touch the knees with your chin. Hold your breath and this position for ten seconds.

2. Let go of your knees and rest your head in the floor. Relax your shoulders and breathe in deeply.

Repeat this movement two or three times.

These are some great stretching exercises that will help you warm up and get ready to start with the Asanas. I emphasized in your breathing and the focus of your attention because this is also a preparation for the Asanas in which you have to do this.

Standing Asanas

All standing positions strengthen your muscles, leg joints and backbone. When you practice these Asanas continually the force and mobility of the back, hips, knees, neck and shoulders will augment significantly. These are invigorating postures that replenish the body and the mind eliminating tensions and ailments.

Standing Asanas tone the entire cardiovascular system, stimulate digestion, regulate the kidneys and relieve constipation. When you practice standing Asanas you will learn how to move correctly; this is basic for other Asanas and yoga sequences, but also for your everyday life. This standing poses will help you get consciousness of the correct way to sit, stand and walk.

Tadasana

In Sanskrit "tada" means mountain and "asana", as you already know, means posture. Tadasana is the Mountain Pose and teaches you to stand firm and erect as a mountain. This position may seem simple but is the base for the rest of the standing Asanas. The mountain posture helps you balance and align the body correctly, bringing firmness, strength, calm and stability to your entire being.

Instructions

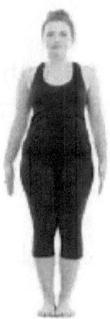

1. Stand up with your back completely extended. Bring your feet together, spreading and stretching the toes of each foot as much as you can.
2. Elevate the internal arches of your feet and press the floor with your metatarsus.
3. Keep the ankles aligned. Contract your quadriceps and keep your knees looking to the front.
4. Put the weight of your body on the heels of your feet until you can distribute all the weight equally on the entire bottom of your feet.
5. Tighten your hips and keep your back straight. Don't tense the upper part of your body.
6. Expand your chest horizontally. Shoulders should be slightly backwards and relaxed.
7. Your arms have to be straight lying at the sides of your thighs. Hand fingers should be all together.
9. Neck has to be straight and centered.
10. Relax your eyes and look straight to the front. Relax all your facial muscles, your tongue and your throat.
11. Remain silent and calmed. Breathe in deeply through your nose and exhale through your mouth. Center your attention in your back and the present.

Vrksasana

"Vrksasana" means tree, so this asana is called the Tree Pose because the whole body stretches upwards simulating to be a tree. This posture improves coordination between the mind and body. Vrksasana also strengthens the back, the ankles and the muscles of the calves and thighs. It helps you achieve balance in your body and even relieves sciatica.

Instructions

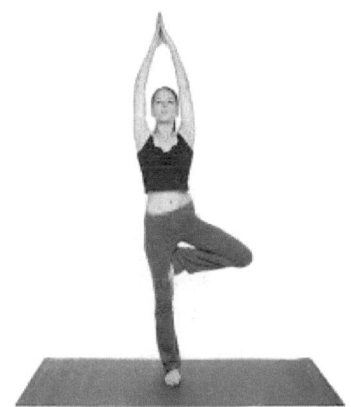

1. Stand up straight and bring your feet together. Breathe in deeply through your nose and exhale through your mouth.
2. Move the weight of your whole body to the left foot. Feel the floor with this foot, focus in what you are doing and get ready to maintain balance.
3. Lift your right foot. Bend your right leg, placing the sole of your foot over your left thigh.
4. Press the right foot against your left thigh as you stretch upwards.
5. Lift your arms over your head and bring your palms together. When you feel comfortable, elevate your arms towards the sky. Hold this position for thirty seconds, if you can't do it, practice until you can.
6. Repeat the same steps but change position of legs.

Utthita Trikonasana

Utthita means, extended, stretched. "Tri" means three and "Kona" means angle, so this asana is called the Extended Triangle Pose. This asana helps expand your chest, augments mobility of the hip joints and neck, stretches, tones and strengthens the back muscles and also helps the hip and calves.

Instructions

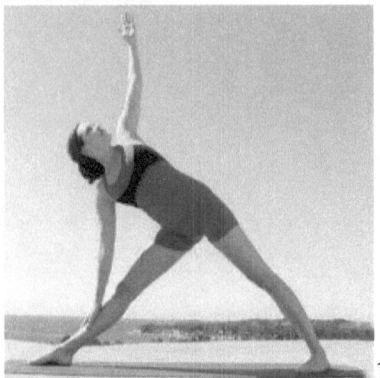

1. Start this pose with Tadasana (Mountain Pose). Breathe in deeply through your nose and exhale through the mouth and spread your legs apart (about 3 or 4 feet).
2. Extend your arms on the sides and make sure they are parallel to the floor and your palms should be facing down.
3. Twirl your right foot outwards in a 90° angle. Now, move your left foot 30 ° inwards. Both toes have to be aligned.
4. Tighten the muscles of your right thigh and move it a bit outwards.
5. Now, start bending your body to the left and make sure both sides of your upper body are completely straight.
6. Push the left side of your hip slightly forward and stretch the coccyx towards your ankle.
7. Place your right hand in the ankle, calf or if you can on the floor. Extend your left arm upwards.
8. Keep your head in neutral position.
9. Breathe in deeply through your nose and exhale through the mouth. Relax, feel your body stretching and center all your attention in what you are doing, in the present.

Utthita Parsvakonasana

"Utthita" means extended, stretched; "Parsva" means flank, side; "Kona" means angle. This is the Extended Side Angle Pose. This is a dynamic and powerful asana and its purpose is to stretch completely the inner thigh and the spine. This pose reinforces the sense of triangulation, expansion and body alignment.

Instructions

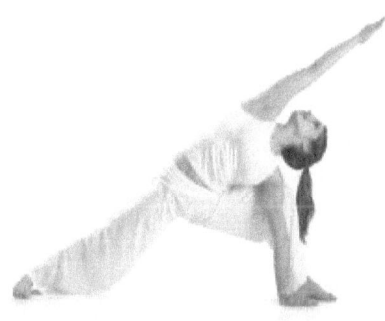

1. Stand in Tadasana. Breathe in deeply and exhale through your mouth.
2. Twirl your right foot 90 ° to the right and keep your left foot facing to the front. Make sure your feet are aligned; the heel of your right foot has to be in the same line with the arch of the left foot.
3. Put your arms in front of you and keep them aligned with your shoulders, palms facing down. Extend and stretch your arms and spread your fingers apart.
4. Bend your right knee until the calf and the thigh form a straight angle. Your knee has to be aligned with the ankle and the left thigh has to be parallel with the floor.
5. Place your right elbow over the knee and the left hand over your hip. Make a pause; watch your posture and breathe in deeply through your nose and exhale through your mouth.
6. Tighten your pelvis and your legs. Slightly move your left thigh backwards and hold it still. Move the right femur forward and stretch the coccyx towards the left foot. Keep doing this as you maintain this posture.
7. Extend the left arm over your left ear. Keep the shoulder integrated.

8. Place the elbow on your leg and keep your head aligned with your back. Stretch your neck and relax.
9. When you feel comfortable maintaining this position, with the elbow on your knee, try to go down and to put your fingers in front or behind the foot.
10. Stretch your sides, your back, your spine and incline backwards to open the posture completely.
11. Breathe in deeply and maintain this pose for thirty seconds. Repeat the same posture twirling the feet to the opposite side.

Virabhadrasana I

Virahabdra was a hero that Siva created, and it makes reference to the inner and spiritual warrior we all have inside. This asana strengthens the legs, stretches the thighs and ankles, improves digestion and develops focus and concentration.

Instructions

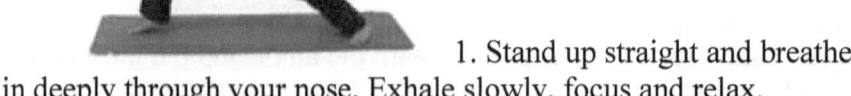

1. Stand up straight and breathe in deeply through your nose. Exhale slowly, focus and relax.
2. Move your left leg forward and bend it in a 90 ° angle. Your left leg has to be straight backwards, and the sole of your foot has to be lying flat on the floor.
3. Extend your arms in front of you, palms facing each other.
4. Bring your hands together and lift your arms pointing to the sky.
5. Tighten your hips and move them slightly forward.
6. Hold this position for thirty seconds breathing in deeply through your nose and exhaling slowly through your mouth. Breathing has to be deep, calmed and comfortable.
Lastly, change sides and repeat the entire sequence.

Virabhadrasana II

This is a variation of the Warrior Pose; it's Virabhadrasana II. This posture strengthens your inner thighs, the chest, the lungs and shoulders. It helps you stretch the legs and ankles and stimulates the abdominal organs. The Warrior Pose II improves digestion and stamina.

Instructions

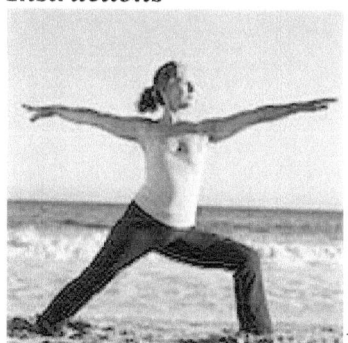

1. Stand up straight and breathe in deeply through your nose. Exhale slowly, focus and relax.

2. Move your left leg forward and bend it in a 90 ° angle. Your left leg has to be straight backwards and the sole of your foot has to be lying flat on the floor.
3. Elevate your left arm in front of you and elevate you right arm in the back. Palms should be facing down, and you have to make sure they are parallel to the floor.
4. Look straight ahead of you and slightly rotate your hips to the front.
5. Relax your shoulders and put them down. Maintain this position for thirty seconds breathing in deeply through your nose and exhaling slowly through your mouth. Your breathing has to be smooth and calmed.
Change sides and repeat this exercise.

Adho Muka Svanasana

"Adho" means down; "Mukha" means face, and "Svana" means dog. This asana resembles a dog stretching with the head and front paws down and the back paws up; this is why is called Downward-Facing Dog. This posture dispels fatigue and brings back the lost energy. It-s indicated for people that suffer from nervous and anxiety attacks and also for the people that get tired quickly. It helps relieve menopause symptoms and premenstrual syndrome, especially when it's done supporting the head on the floor.

Instructions

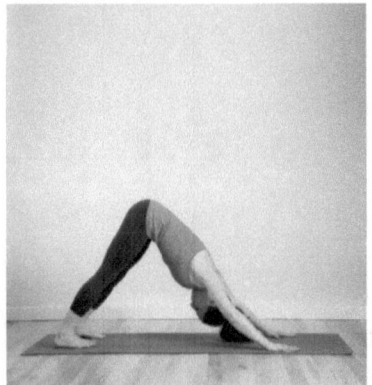

1. Place your knees and hands on the floor. Make sure your knees are directly under your hips, and the hands should be placed in front of your shoulders. Spread the fingers of your hands and leave both indexes parallel to each other.
2. Inhale deeply as you bend your toes forward, supporting yourself on them. Lift your knees from the floor as you exhale. You have to feel all the weight of your body in your hands. The heels of your feet have to be slightly separated from the floor.
3. Once you are up, distribute your weight equally between your hands and your legs. Elevate your hips so that your coccyx points to the sky.
4. With a deep exhale, press the back part of your thighs backwards and bring the heels of your feet back to the floor. Stretch your knees.
5. Stretch your arms from the wrist all the way to the shoulders and keep your head between your arms aligning it with your back.
6. Move your shoulders back so that the upper part of your back forms a straight line with the arms. Your body will be forming an inverted V.

7. Maintain this posture for about three minutes as you breathe deeply and are conscious of your body and posture.
These are some standing Asanas you can start practicing right away. They are for beginners, and you need to work and master them to be able to move to some more advanced positions.

Sitting Asanas

Sitting Asanas give elasticity to the hips, knees, ankles and inguinal muscles. Eliminate tension and stiffness in the diaphragm and throat soothing and facilitating breathing. These postures hold firmly the spinal column, easing the mind and stretching the muscles of the heart. Blood circulation is improved in all parts of the body. These are key poses, because when you master them you can maintain the body relaxed during meditation or the practice of Pranayamas.

Sukasana (The Easy Pose)

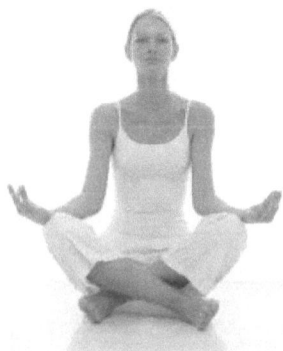

1. Sit on the floor extending your legs; cross them in the position you feel more comfortable in.
2. Center your attention in the back and make sure it's completely straight.
3. Your chest has to be elevated, the shoulders relaxed and naturally thrown back.
4. Stretch your neck and make sure your chin is parallel with the floor.

You will note that with these postures the lower and nearer the knees are to the floor, the straighter the back will be. When you are a beginner you will have to pay close attention in keeping your back straight. The process of gradually pressing the knees against the floor is very beneficial for your joints; augments force and flexibility and help with arthritis.

Padmasana (Lotus Pose)

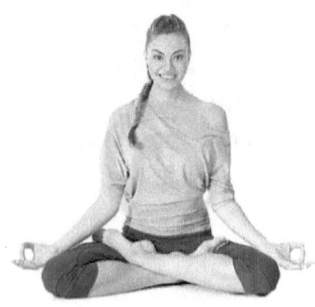

1. Sit on the floor or blanket and extend your legs forward.
2. Lift and bend your left foot and put it on top of your right thigh.
3. Now, put the right foot on top of the left thigh. The right leg always has to be on top.
This position straightens your back automatically and favors a deep meditation.

Ardha Padmasana (Half Lotus Pose)

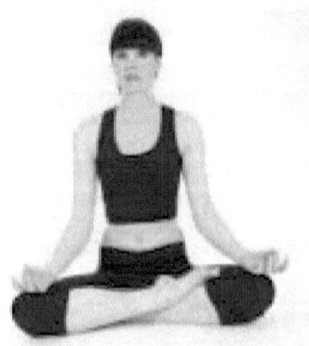

1. Sit down on the floor and extend your legs in front of you.

2. Bend you right foot and pose it on top of the right thigh; as high as possible. Your left heel should be on top of the right heel.
3. The knees have to be on the floor with the heels directly one on top of the other.
Alternate legs, this way you develop the same flexibility in both knees and sides of the hips.

Vajrasana (The Rock Pose)

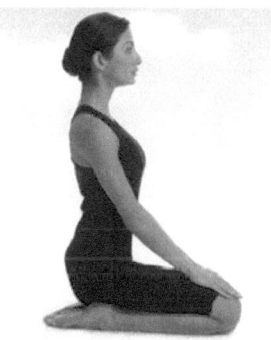

1. Kneel down on the floor or over a blanket to feel comfortable.
2. Sit down on top of your heels. The tips of your feet have to be flat on the floor.
It's called the Rock Pose for its positive effects on digestion, which allows you to "eat rocks".

Virasana (Hero Pose)

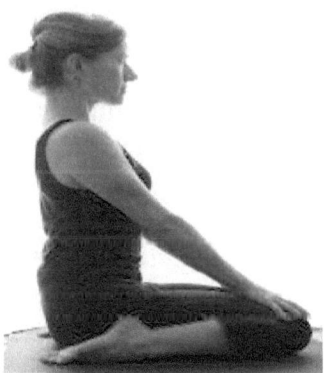

1. Kneel down on the floor.
2. Open your feet and sit down in between.

This posture canalizes sexual energy.

Savasana (The Corpse Pose)

This is not a sitting position but I have to include it, since t's a
neutral and essential position in yoga practice. It's very simple and
it's a pose that will help you relax and find your center and balance.
It's used when you are starting some other Asanas and for some
sequences.

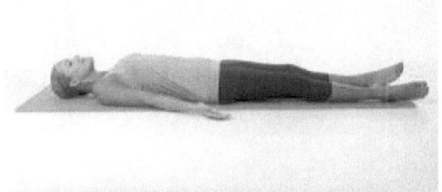

1. Lie down on the floor and slightly spread your legs apart. Your
toes have to be twirled towards opposite your inner thighs.
2. Place your arms away from the rest of your body; not much, but in
a middle distance.
3. Relax your neck and close your eyes.
4. Center your attention in your body and breathe normally.
5. Move your attention to every part of your body; one part at a time.
Keep your mind focused on relaxation.
Keep this position as long as you want and feel comfortable.

Forward Bending Asanas

These are the Asanas, in which the trunk leans forward, curving the
spinal column and stretching the back. These postures induce to
reflection and calm.
Bending Asanas compress the abdominal organs and relax them.
This generates a singular effect over the nervous system, refreshing
the brain and regulating blood circulation. With these yoga positions,
tension in the organs is eliminated, and the senses rest. The
suprarenal glands are also relieved and work more efficiently.
The bending postures stimulate the liver and kidneys and improve
digestion. Practicing these postures reduces tension and helps with

insomnia. Given that the body is in a horizontal position during this bends, the heart is under less stress because it doesn't have to pump blood against gravity and blood circulates better through-out the body. These Asanas bring physical and emotional firmness and balance; they are great for calming the mind.

Paschimottanasana (The Forward Bend)

Paschimottanasana means "intense stretch to the west" but we call it the Forward Bend. In this pose, all the upper part of your body is intensely stretched and posing the forehead in the legs soothes the frontal brain. It causes a truly magical effect over your mind; when you are altered or stressed it gives you peace by restoring the nervous system. It tones the kidneys, bladder and pancreas,activates the liver and digestive system. This position also calms headaches and anxiety and reduces fatigue.

Instructions

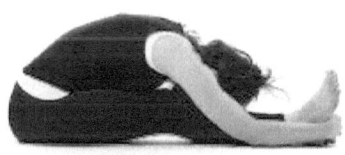

1. Sit on the floor bringing your legs together and extending them as much as you can. Your back has to be completely straight.
2. Place your hands on the floor beside your hips. Your fingers have to be pointing in the same direction of the feet. Push your hands against the floor stretching your spine and the trunk upwards.
3. As you inhale, raise your arms above the head until they form a perfect line with your trunk. Stretch as much as you can, do it as if you were trying to touch the sky.
4. As you exhale, bring all your upper body and arms towards your legs; **bending by the hips**. While you are descending keep your

back straight and place your abdomen on the thighs. At the end of the exhalation grab your toes with both hands.

5. Try to make your head touch the knees (or as close as possible). Breathing has to be soft and if you can, rest your elbows on the floor.

6. Hold this position for thirty seconds and then when you inhale, move back to an upright position keeping the back and arms completely stretched and straight.

Repeat this exercise at least two more times, you will feel great.

Uttanasana (Standing Forward Bend)

In Sanskrit the word "Ut" means intense and "Tan" means stretch, so this is an intense stretching pose. This is a basic posture that is used between other standing Asanas to rest. When you bring your head down the blood flow to the brain is increased, and this produces a sensation of well-being. This posture oxygenates the central nervous system, alleviates physical and mental fatigue and rejuvenates the spinal nerves and cerebral cells.

Instructions

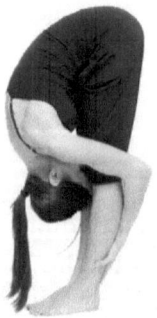

1. Stand in Tadasana position and elevate your arms to the front.

2. Exhale and bend your body forward **from the hips**, not the waist. You have to stretch your frontal torso.

3. If it's possible, with the knees are completely straight, put your fingers or your palms on the floor. If you can't do this just go as low as you can; don't force anything.

4. Now, if you can put the palms of your hands on the back of your legs, on the ankles. If you can't do this, cross your arms in front of you and hold your elbows.
5. With every inhale, stretch your frontal trunk as much as you can. Let your head relax completely.
6. Hold this posture for thirty seconds or one minute if you can.

Janu Sirsasana (The Head-To-Knee Forward Bend Pose)

In Sanskrit, the word knee is said "janu" and head is translated as "sirsa". This position exerts a tremendous dynamic impact over the body and brings many benefits. This pose teaches you how to let go and free tension from the mind and the body. It stretches the calves muscles, lower back, shoulders and inner thighs. Janu Sirsasana tones the abdominal organs and aids with high blood pressure, insomnia, fatigue, headache and sinusitis.

Instructions

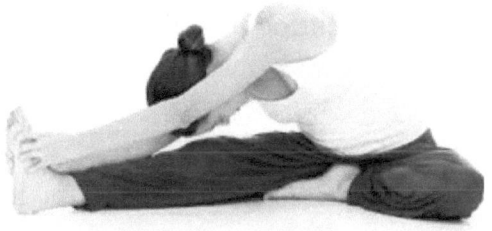

1. Sit on the floor with your legs completely extended.
2. Bend your right leg and place the heel on your left thigh. Press the instep against the floor. Your right knee has to be as close to the floor as possible, and has to create a 90 ° angle with the other leg. Keep your left leg as stretched as you can.
3. Bring your hands to the thighs and as you do this push your glutei backwards. Root your legs to the floor, tighten your muscles and keep them like this during the whole posture. Make sure your right gluteus doesn't separate from the floor.
4. Inhale deeply through your nose and as you exhale slowly bend forward over your left leg. Bring your hand to the foot; if you can't reach the foot then stop where you feel comfortable.

5. Inhale and be conscious of your posture, your breathing; soothe and relax.

6. Try to twirl your trunk a little more towards the leg that is extended, so that your sternum is directly on top of the leg. Keep both shoulders at the same height.

7. Keep all the strength in your legs and pelvis. With every exhale, extend more and more over the stretched leg.

8. Hold this position as much as you can, at least one minute. Make sure you don't arch your back during this posture. Focus in bringing your chest to the thigh, instead of focusing in bringing your head to the knee.

Ardha Kurmasana (Half Tortoise Pose)

In Sanskrit, the word "kurma" means tortoise and "ardha" means half; this is why this pose is called the Half Tortoise Pose. This yoga posture improves lung functioning and is beneficial for people that suffer from asthma and lung diseases. This pose also improves digestion and helps with constipation. With its continuous practice it gives you clarity of mind, and eliminates tension from the back and neck.

Instructions

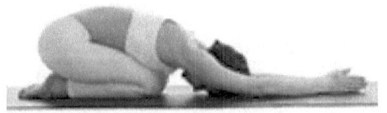

1. Kneel on the floor or a yoga mat. Your glutei have to be on top of your heels.

2. Bring your feet and knees together and keep your back completely extended.

3. Place the palms of your hands in front of you on the floor. Inhale deeply through your nose.

4. As you exhale start bending forward **by the wais**t; sliding your hands slowly on the floor. You have to put your chest on your thighs, and your head has to be perfectly aligned with your spine.
5. Relax the shoulders and rest your forehead comfortably on the floor.
6. Stretch your arms as much as you can and hold this position at least for one minute.

Extension Asanas

These Asanas are perfect for beginners and you can start feeling better right away!
Extension Asanas are the ones in which the trunk bend forward and the thorax expands. In these postures the spinal column makes an extension movement, stimulating nervous roots and strengthening the back.
These Asanas charge your body with energy and are very useful for people with depression. They open the chest and give flexibility to the spine. Arms and shoulders become stronger, improved physical and mental attention. Extension Asanas allow more cell oxygenation and optimize respiratory functions. They have a rejuvenating and invigorating effect.

Bhujangasana (The Cobra Pose)

This posture produces an important effect over the spinal column due to its back flexion. Rejuvenates and stimulates the nervous system.

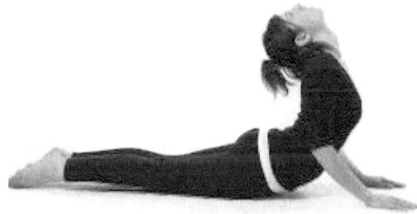

1. Lie down over your belly and extend your arms in front of you.

2. Rest your head over your arms and regulate your breathing. You should inhale and exhale calmly, constantly bringing oxygen into your blood.

3. Slowly lift your head and look towards the sky. Move your arms placing your hands behind the shoulders. Allow your chest to support your weight.

4. Straighten your elbows gently, pushing the upper part of your body from the floor. Lift your chest and center the weight of your body on the stomach.

5. Stretch your arms completely and slightly twirl those inwards. Relax your back and support your weight with both arms.

6. Breathe in deeply and every time you exhale try to lift your chest even more. Keep your shoulders down.

Hold this position for thirty seconds and repeat three times.

Matsyasana (The Fish Pose)

The fish pose exerts amazing effects over the thyroid glands. Breathing is enhanced and the lungs get cleaned and stimulated. This position reliefs many respiratory ailments.

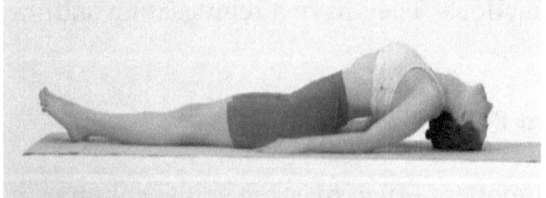

1. Lie down on your back keeping your feet together.

2. Put your arms on the sides and rest your palms on the floor. Relax and breathe in deeply through your nose and then slowly exhale through your mouth.

3. Bring your hands under your bottom. Arch your back and let your head hang and rest on the floor.

4. Hold this position for thirty seconds and make sure you only arch your back; the rest of your body has to be tightened and your head needs to be completely relaxed.

Twisting Asanas

These Asanas are characterized by the twirl of the spinal column. The back twist can be made from multiple positions, and sometimes the twirl is combined with other movements. These postures mainly massage the abdominal organs, strengthen the spine and balance the nervous system.

During the twists, the pelvic organs are compressed and charged with energy. They improve diaphragm flexibility and alleviate hip ailments. These Asanas increase the blood flow to the spinal nerves, toning internal organs, augmenting energy levels and giving peace of mind. These twists are very effective in calming back pain, headaches and stiffness of the neck and shoulders. While the trunk is twisting, the kidneys and abdominal organs activate and improve digestion and eliminate tiredness.

Vakrasana (The Twisted Pose)

The word "vakra" in Sanskrit means twisted, for this its name in English. This pose is also called Marichyasana in honor of Marichy, grandfather of Surya, god of the sun.

This pose gives great flexibility to the spine, stretches and revitalizes every dorsal muscle avoiding tension and frayed nerves. Induces to deep relaxation sedating the nervous system and massages all the organs from the abdominal cavity. This pose also combats stiffness in muscle and legs and regulates renal function.

Instructions

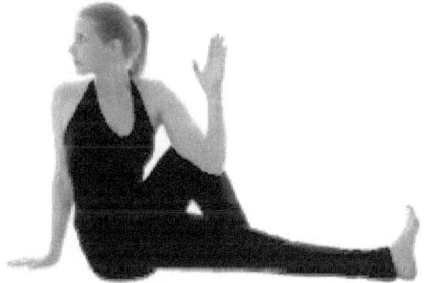

1. Sit on the floor or yoga mat and extend your legs.
2. Bring your inner thighs inwards and push your glutei backwards to stretch your back completely.

3. Extend your right leg and bend the left leg. The sole of your left foot has to be lying flat on the floor beside your right knee.
4. Place the fingers of your right hand on the floor beneath the gluteus.
5. Stop for an instant and control your breathing. Inhale deeply and as you do this stretch your back and root your glutei to the floor.
6. Bring your left hand to your left knee. Exhale and twist your trunk towards the right side of your body. Start twisting from the waist up and use your hands and arms to help you do this.
7. Gently place your left elbow on the left knee. Keep your back straight at all times.
8. The head is the last thing that twirls; the neck has to follow the spine's direction and doesn't have to be forced. Move your chin a bit up, look above your shoulder but don't force the posture.
9. Breath in deeply ten times; make sure your breathing is relaxed, profound and calmed. Don't hold your breath.
Repeat the same steps but now to the other side.

Jathara Parivartanasana (The Revolved Abdomen Pose)

In Sanskrit "Jathara" means abdomen and "parivrta" means twisted. This pose acts over the hip joints, stretches the glutei muscles and exerts a soft pressure in the abdomen.

Instructions

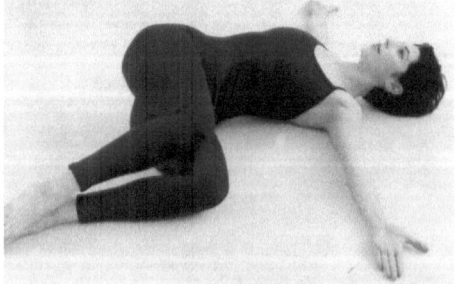

1. Lie down on your back with the arms extended in a horizontal position in line with the shoulders.
2. Bend your knees bringing your feet towards the hips. The soles of your feet have to be flat on the floor.

3. Twist your knees towards the left side of your body until the left knee touches the floor. Your left thigh and knee are on top of your left knee and thigh, and your shoulders should be flat on the floor.
4. Hold this posture and feel how your inner thighs, arms, neck, stomach and back stretch. With every exhale relax more and more. Repeat the same steps to work on the other side of your body.

Ardha Matsyendrasana (The Half Lord of the Fishes Pose)

The word "ardha" means half and "matsyendrasana" means king of the fish. The name given to this pose is in honor to Matsyendra, one of the first teachers of Hatha Yoga. This posture gives elasticity to the back, augments appetite and digestive power, and helps heal nervous disorders. It's also recommended to augment vitality and to obtain mental peace.

Instructions

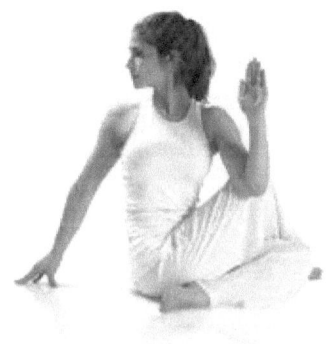

1. Sit on the floor with your back straight and your legs together and extended.
2. Bend your left leg and put your heel underneath your right thigh. Keep it as close to your glutcus as you can.
3. Bring the sole of your right foot to the floor beside and outside your left knee.
4. Place your right hand on the floor beneath the gluteus.

5. Move your left arm over the right knee and place it on the outer part of your right leg. Now, grab your right foot or ankle with the left hand.
6. Inhale stretching upwards and when you exhale twist the trunk to the right as much as possible.
7. Finally, when the head is completely twisted look over your shoulder, and bring your left elbow on top of the knee.
Don't force your posture, relax, breathe in deeply and after one minute of holding the pose repeat the same instructions to work on the other side of your body.

Chapter 6: Sun Salutation

Sun Salutation is a series of twelve easy and simple Asanas that bring elasticity and massage every organ of your organism. This sequence is considered as one of the most complete yoga exercises that exist. The reason that is so effective is for the combination of its Asanas with conscious breathing, that leave the body, the mind, and spirit relaxed and alert.
In a general way, we can say that Sun Salutation strengthens every system in the organism, potentiating health, physical, mental and spiritual energy. Every posture has its own finality, but together they are an amazing gift for your organism.

Sun Salutation Benefits
-Improves muscles and joints flexibility
-Strengthens the loco-motor apparatus
-Brings focus, calm, serenity and inner force
-Stimulates blood circulation
-Detoxifies the organism
-Strengthens the heart
-Balances the chakras
-Alleviates depression, anxiety and stress
-Stimulates self-healing
-Prepares you to affront life with enthusiasm, joy and serenity

Tips before Getting Started

Sunrise

Sun Salutation can be made at any time of the day, but I advise that you do it in the morning when you wake up. Try to practice it before you do anything else; just when you wake up, before having breakfast. It will not take a lot of time, with ten minutes is more than enough to feel the benefits.

Space
Designate a special place in your house; it can be a room, the garden, wherever you feel more comfortable. Make sure you have enough space to move freely.

Focus
It's very important that no one or nothing distracts you. An important factor in Sun Salutation is to potentiate, besides the body, also your mind, focus and concentration in whatever you are doing; in the present.

Take it Slowly
Remember that yoga is not a competitive sport and you don't have to do it perfect the first times you practice. If you have been practicing your Asanas, this should not be complicated for you, but it still takes time to master. Keep practicing patiently and give your body some time.

Consciousness and Rest
When you finish the sequence I advise that you lie down on the floor, in the Corpse Pose or any other position in which you feel completely comfortable. Rest for a while, at least five minutes and normalize your breathing. Take consciousness of your body and your mind.

Discipline
To receive all the benefits this sequence brings, it's important that you make a commitment with yourself. The ideal is to practice this every day without exception. The world is not going to end if for some reason you can't do it, but try to be disciplined and set it as an important goal for you.

Instructions

Pranam Asana (Prayer Pose)

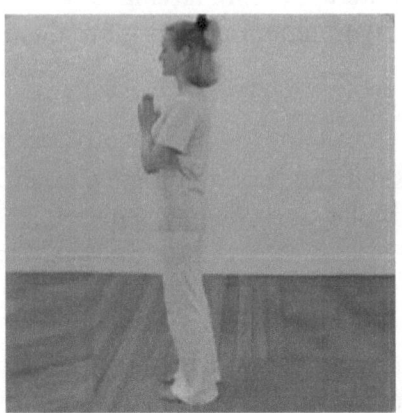

Stand up straight with your feet together. Bring the palms of your hands together in the Prayer Pose. Your hands have to be at the same height of the heart and your weight has to be evenly distributed. Close your eyes and center your attention in your body; empty your mind, clear your thoughts and simply…exist.

Urdhva Hastasana (Raised Arms Pose)

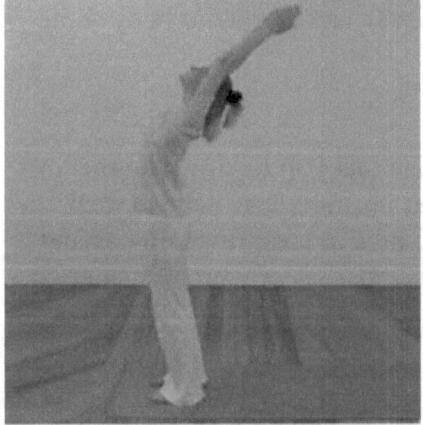

Inhale deeply through your nose and as you do this, extend your arms upwards and stretch them as much as you can. Delicately arch your back and arms backwards and bring your pelvis a bit forward. Elbows and knees have to be entirely stretched and your head has to be situated between the arms and with the chin facing the sky.

Uttanasana (Standing Forward Bend)

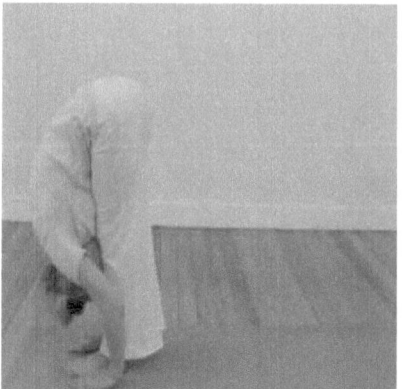

Inhale deeply, and when you exhale bend forward and place your palms on the floor. Try to touch your knees with your head; do it slowly and don't force anything. Your hands have to be in line with your feet and your back should be comfortably extended.

Ashwa Sanchalanasana (Runner Lunge or Equestrian Stretch Pose)

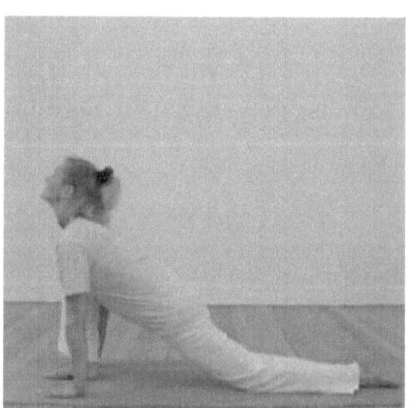

Move your right leg back, as far as you can. Support your right knee on the floor and make sure the tip of your foot faces the sky. Keep your hands on the floor in line with your shoulders. Your left foot has to be exactly in between your arms. Breathe in deeply and as you exhale move your head a bit upwards.

Chaturanga Dandasana (The Plank Pose)

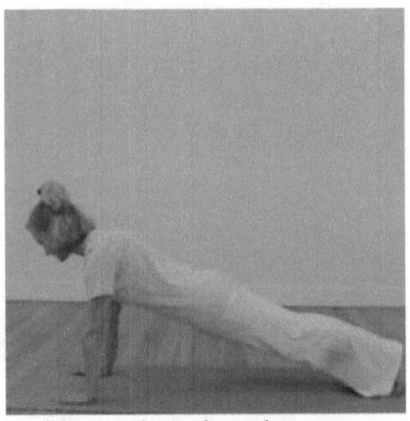

Hold your breath and move your left leg backwards and place it beside your right leg. Move your head down a bit so that it forms a straight line with your back. Keep your knees extended and take a deep breath through your nose. Exhale, and as you do this lower your body. Keep your elbows at your side.

Shisuasana (The Child Pose)

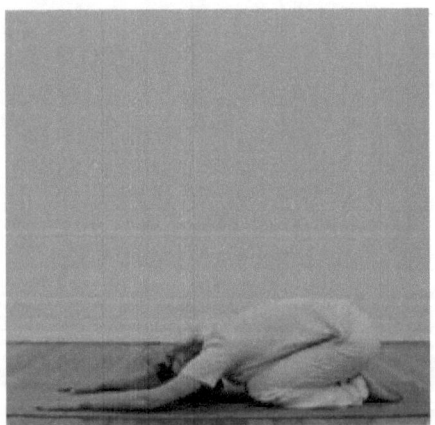

Exhale deeply and move your hips towards your heels. Bring your forehead to the knees and rest it (your forehead) comfortably on the floor. Your hands should be firmly stretched on the floor. Breathe in deeply and center your attention in your body and the present.

Ashtanga Namaskara (Knees-Chest-Chin-Pose)

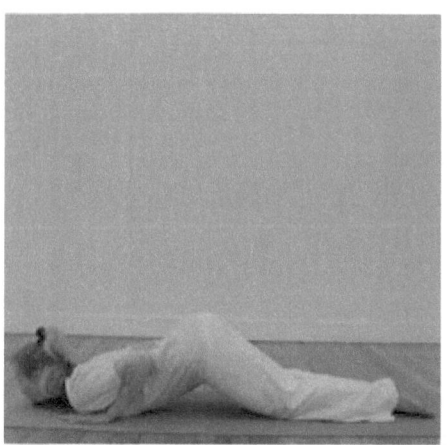

Gently and slowly slide forward, keeping your chin near the floor. Make sure your shoulders are directly above your wrists. Firmly hold your sides with your elbows and point them back towards your heels. Keep your hips lifted off the floor. Bring your chest to the floor and make sure it is situated between your hands. Lastly, put your chin on the floor and be conscious of your body and your posture.

Bhujangasana (The Cobra Pose)

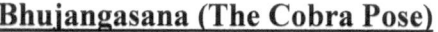

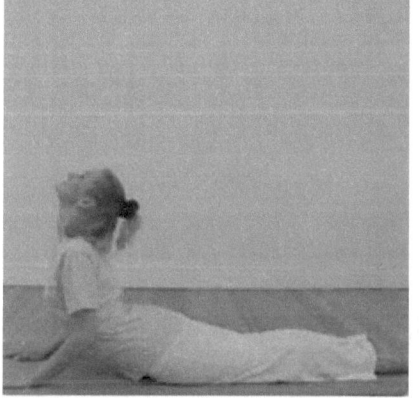

Exhale and move into the cobra pose. Keep your elbows close to your sides and lift your shoulders. Put your pelvis against the floor and move your torso up focusing on the inclination of the upper part of your back. Breathe in deeply and relax.

Adho Muka Svanasana (Downward Facing Dog)

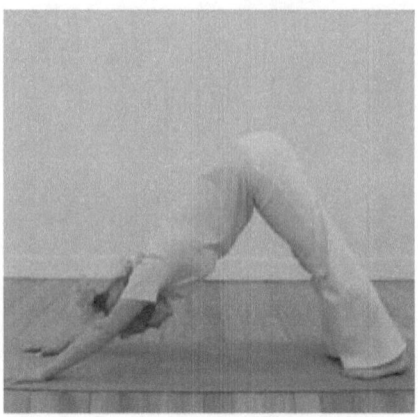

Exhale and put your hands on the ground. Keep your arms completely straight. Raise your hips and place your head in between your arms, making a straight line with your back. Your body has to form an inverted V. Try to lay your soles and heels flat on the floor.

Ashwa Sanchalanasana (Runner Lunge or Equestrian Stretch Pose)

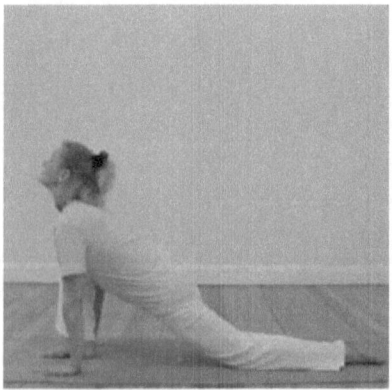

Breathe in deeply and as you do this bring your right foot forward. Keep your knee on the floor and look up. Your left foot has to be facing the sky.

Uttanasana (Standing Forward Bend)

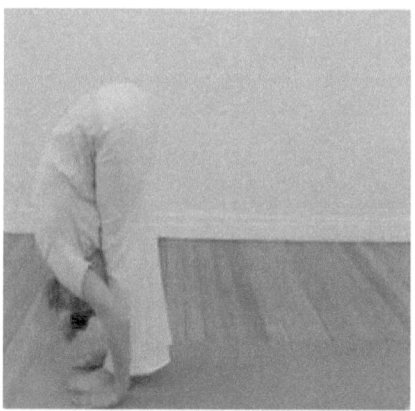

Exhale and move your left foot forward. It has to be aligned with the right foot. Keeping your hands in place, straighten your legs but keep your waist bent and your upper body lowered. Touch your knees with your forehead if you can, and exhale.

Urdhva Hastasana (Raised Arms Pose)

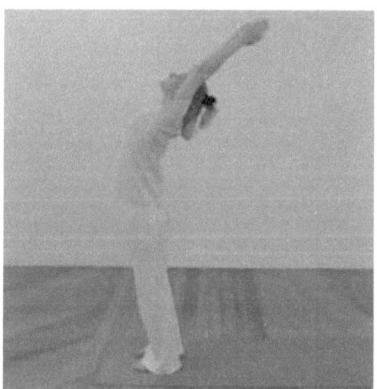

Breathe in deeply and come back to a vertical position. Lift your arms and slightly arch your back, head and arms backwards. Move your pelvis a bit forward and breathe in deeply.

Tadasana (The Mountain Posture)

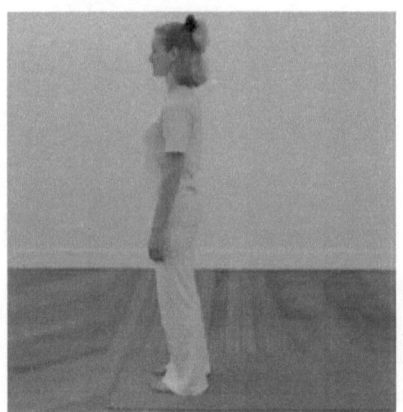

Exhale and lower your arms and place them at the sides of your body. Breathe in deeply through your nose and exhale through your mouth. Feel the difference between both sides of your body. Congratulations! You have successfully completed half of the series of postures of the Sun Salutation sequence. If you want to perform the full sequence repeat from the beginning using the opposite leg you used for this series. I advise you to do this because it's important to maintain balance between both sides of your body.

7. Conclusion

As you already know by now, yoga makes you love yourself just the way you are and accept your body, which is unique and incomparable. But yoga also helps you transcend, making you realize your body is not your only identity. Your body is an infinite being, is part of your ego or your individuality. If you work on it, it's to be stronger, more flexible and to enjoy of better physical and mental health. There's spiritual progression only if the body is healthy, and radiant health opens you a door to a higher level of consciousness. Yoga may start with the body, but it's not a narcissistic practice, frivolous or vain; it's totally the opposite. Yoga teaches you to love yourself, and because of that love, it makes you respect and take care of your body. With the balance between body and mind, health will come automatically, and with it you'll be in better shape. Yoga's purpose is to open you to love, and to teach you, that you don't have to be different to achieve happiness and freedom. Yoga wants you to know the truth; all that you need is already in you; all that you want you have it; everything is inside of you already.

Yoga gives you a strong body, a big spirit and a quiet mind. You don't need to fulfill any requirements to practice yoga; you don't have to be something you are not. You don't have to be thinner, stronger or young; yoga is simple and is universal.

Yoga relates to life in more than a thousand ways; as a fountain of knowledge and life path is a topic to which we can dedicate an eternity. But, as many wise men and masters have said; knowledge, words and formulas are nothing without experience. Comprehension is non-transferrable and impossible to define, so this means everyone will have a unique and special path in yoga.

I hope your journey, which is just starting, is amazing, full of significances, of fantastic experiences, of peace and of inner growth.

8. THANK YOU FOR READING!

Thank You so much for reading this book. If this title gave you a ton of value, It would be amazing for you to leave a REVIEW !

THANK YOU FOR DOWNLOADING! IF YOU ENJOYED THIS BOOK AND WOULD LIKE TO READ MORE TITLES FROM MY COLLECTION CLICK THIS LINK